101 Ways to Date Your Mate

Hundreds of fun & romantic dating ideas

Earl & Rose Smith
(Mr. & Mrs. Romance)

1 0 1   Ways to Date Your Mate

Copyright (c) 1997 by Rose & Earl Smith
Printed in the United States of America.
Published by:

William Havens Publishing
4900 Mesa Bonita Ct. NW
Albuquerque, NM 87120
505-899-3121

Publisher's Cataloging in Publication Data
Smith, Earl, 1967-
Smith, Rose, 1967-
101 Ways to Date Your Mate
1.   Self-help. 2. Psychology. 3. Relationships. 4. How-to. I. Title

This book is available for quantity discounts call 505-899-3121 for more information.

~Table of Contents~

It's A Date!

date (dāt) n. 6 an appointment for a set time esp. with a person of the opposite sex.

When's the last time you really had a fantastic time on a date? Dating is fun & it doesn't have to be expensive. A good date can last anywhere from a couple of hours to a couple of weeks. Whether you're single and looking to date someone, or you've been married for years and you want to date your mate all over again, this book's filled with wonderfully romantic ideas.

If you're single and looking to make a lasting impression on the person of your dreams, you'll knock their socks off with the many ideas in this book. *101 Ways to Date Your Mate* is also ideal for married couples whose marriages are stuck in an unromantic rut. You'll find hundreds of fun ways to get off life's treadmill and enjoy yourselves—and each other again.

Use it to schedule evenings out, & evenings in. Use the 101 + the 50 bonus ideas and make up your own. Bonus love recipes and love

prescriptions are included. And to put hundreds of romance resources at your fingertips, make use of the Romantic Resource sections throughout this book. Use *101 Ways to Date Your Mate* to turn romance into something special!

An Angel's Caress

Angels above, please protect our love...Protect it from indifference,
From taking our loved ones for granted
Feeling we can express our love tomorrow...
For tomorrow will always come.
Please send angels to caress our love & wrap it
in a blanket of warmth, caring and understanding,
Help us learn to share the love we feel from an angel's warm touch.
Help us share those same feelings with our loved ones.
For in this world filled with hate, fear, violence and indifference,
We sometimes forget about the sheer beauty of our love..
Let the caress of the angels always remind us that we've been given a
precious gift ...
The gift of love.

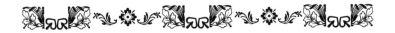

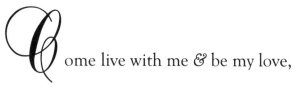

ome live with me & be my love,

And we will some new pleasures prove

Of golden sands and crystal brooks,

with silken lines & silver hooks.

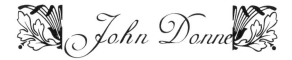

John Donne

Who says pull never gets you anywhere? If love tugs at your heartstrings, you're sitting on top of the world.

Burton Hillis

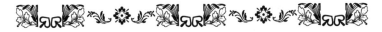

Musical Notes ♪♪♫♪..

1

Sing It Out Loud--Call your partner's answering machine on the job (when you know he or she won't be there to pick up) and leave a singing message. Sing Stevie Wonder's song *I Just Called To Say I Love You*. Add your own lyrics asking your mate for a date.

2

Let's Go Dancing—This is one of the first things to go once a couple 'settles down' and gets married. Yet, it's one of the most fun activities you can share, if both of you enjoy dancing.(Make a promise that you will *never* 'settle down' when you're married or in a long-term relationship—just make sure to share all the passion and the good times with your partner.)

3

Slow Dance On Your Favorite Song—If you don't like dancing in public, or even if you do, dance together in private.

4

Slow Dance On Your Partner's Favorite Song—If you're out in public, ask the band to play your partner's favorite song.

5

Private serenade—Go out to a restaurant with a singer & secretly ask the host or hostess to have the singer serenade your love. Earl took me to one of our favorites restaurants and had the waitress, who was a part-time performer, sing a beautiful ballad, called *Nothing's Going To Harm You.* It was a moment that was so unique and special it brought tears to my eyes.

6

Buy a Special Music Box–When you're out on a special date or romantic holiday together, buy your partner a special music box that plays a love melody–the two of you will always think of the wonderful time you shared together when you hear the music.

7

Sending You My Love–Send your mate a singing telegram asking for a special date.

8

Have a Private Concert—Curl up on the couch together one afternoon or evening, and listen to your favorite music be it classical or contemporary. You can even have a special tape or CD made for your mate to celebrate any special occasion, wedding, anniversary, Valentine's Day, etc. The song is sung by a famous artist and your mate will receive the sheet music. The price starts at $24.95. Call P.S. I Love You at 1-800-725-SONG.

❤❧❤Romantic Resources❤❧❤

Favorite Love Songs:

Timeless Classics

Unforgettable, Nat King Cole
The First Time Ever I Saw Your Face, Roberta Flack
Ain't No Mountain High Enough, Diana Ross
Strangers In The Night, Frank Sinatra
Memories, Elvis Presley
Georgia On My Mind, Ray Charles
My Eyes Adore You, Frankie Valle
Killing Me Softly, Roberta Flack
Love Is A Many Splendored Thing
Could It Be Magic, Barry Manilow

Pop/Contemporary

Soul Provider, Michael Bolton
Hello, Lionel Richie
Three Times A Lady, Commodores
We've Only Just Begun, The Carpenters
Evergreen, Barbara Striesand
Find One Hundred Ways, Quincy Jones (Sung by James Ingram)
Just The Way You Are, Billy Joel
I Love You, Olivia Newton John
I Will Always Love You, Whitney Houston

I Just Called To Say I Love You, Stevie Wonder
Color My World, Chicago
On Bended Knee, Boyz II Men
It's Our Anniversary, Toni, Tone, Tony
All My Loving, The Beatles
You Are My Lady, Freddy Jackson

Soul

Baby, Baby, Baby, TLC
My Girl, The Temptations
Living For The Love Of You, Isley Brothers
Best Of My Love, The Emotions
Breathe Again, Toni Braxton
Forever My Lady, Jodeci
Slow Hands, The Pointer Sisters
Turn Off The Lights, Teddy Pendagrass

Country

Lady, Kenny Rogers
If I Don't Love You, Grits Ain't Groceries, George Jones
I Swear, John Michael Montgomery
Bop, Dan Seals
She Believes in Me, Kenny Rogers
Faith in Me, Faith in You, Doug Stone
Your Love Amazes Me, John Berry
The Love You Gave to Me, Tanya Tucker

New Age

Down to the Moon, Andreas Vollenwieder
Heartsounds, David Lanz
Winter Into Spring, George Winston
Forever Friends, Justo Almario
Solid Colors, Liz Story
Wintersong, Paul Winter
Childhood & Memory, William Ackerman
A Winter's Solstice, Windham Hill Artists

Yanni, Reflections Of Passion

Love Songs With a Rockin' Beat

She Loves You, The Beatles
Just A Touch Of Love, C+C Music Factory
Show Me Love, Robin S.
All My Loving, The Beatles

Still A Thrill, Jody Whatley
Let's Get Physical, Olivia Newton John
Some Kind Of Lover, Jody Whatley
I Want To Rock With You, Michael Jackson

Gift Resources For Music Lovers:

Noteworthy Music: Their catalog has 12,000 CDs from classical, big band, country and rock: 603-881-5729

. . . when we find ourselves

In the place just right

It will be in the valley

Of love and delight.

from "Simple Gifts"

a Shaker Hymn

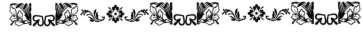

All play & all play make

Jack & Jill...uh

Smile.

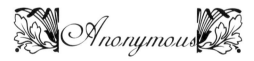

Anonymous

Come Play With Me

9

𝓛aughter (mixed with a little love) Really Is The Best Medicine—
When your partner is having a bad day or going through
a difficult time because of job or life hassles, buy a humorous little pick
me up gift or humorous card designed to make your partner laugh at his
or her troubles. Give it to your partner and be there to talk, hold,
console or listen.

⌊10⌋

❧ Queen/King For a Day–Your mate's wish is your command. This one's fun to do for a birthday, anniversary, mother's day, father's day, or just because.

⌊11⌋

❧ The Treasure Hunt–Send your mate on a treasure hunt for a present. Leave stick on notes on refrigerators, mirrors, or doors leading to the present. Have one last note wrapped inside the present leading straight to you. Be waiting for your partner with relaxing drinks and snacks. Use the time to unwind and be together.

⌊12⌋

❧ Sportsplay–Go out to a basketball court and play ball, go play tennis, or go bowling. Play any sport you both enjoy.

⌊13⌋

❧ Football Widow–NOT!–Buy two tickets to your favorite sporting event and take your mate with you.

⟍14⟋

❧ Take a Class Together—Take a hobby class, a class on car maintenance, or any life-skill class you'd both be interested in and go together.

⟍15⟋

❧ Getting to Know You—*Getting to Know You* is a fun book filled with 365 questions to help you get to know your mate even better. Available in most gift stores or call World Leisure Corporation at 1-617-569-1966. The Getting To Know You Better two-person board game also helps you learn more about each other. Order from Seasons catalog. Call 1-800-776-9677, or write P.O. Box 64545, Saint Paul, Minnesota, 55164.

⟍16⟋

❧ Take Your Mate on a Mystery Date—Make all the arrangements. Earl took me to a bed and breakfast in New Mexico out in the country. He arranged for the sitter, took three days off in the middle of the week, packed the bags, and whisked me off for a romantic mid-week holiday I'll never forget.

⌐17⌐

♀ Have an Enchanted Evening–Play *An Enchanted Evening*. It's a board game created by a husband and wife couple in San Francisco. You can pick it up at most toy or game stores, or you can write to Games Partnership Ltd., 116 New Montgomery, Suite 500, San Francisco, California 94105.

⌐18⌐

♀ Surprise!–Plan a surprise party for your mate for any occasion~birthday, anniversary or just because. Save a special private gift for your private celebration.

⌐19⌐

♀ Amuse Me–Go out to a local amusement park together~without the kids. You'll have a ball together.

⌐20⌐

♀ Play "I'd like to get to know you"–Go to a party or outing in separate cars and act like you just met. One couple played this scenario for all it's worth. They went to a party where most of the people attending were co-workers of his and most had never met his 'date'. When she walked in looking very sexy, he told his friends that he wanted to get to know her. They didn't think he had a chance. He walked over, introduced himself, danced with her and proceeded to 'win her over.' His buddies stood there with gaped mouths when she left the party with him.

21

❧ Rub a Dub—Two lovers in the tub—Make a date to take a bubble-bath together. Relax and have fun.

22

❧ Play An Affair To Remember—Pretend you are having an affair with your partner. In *Sizzling Monogamy*, we talk about how to have a romantic marital affair with your spouse. This technique kept us monogamous during a year-long separation forced by Earl's military duties. *Sizzling Monogamy* sells for $12.95 and you can pick it up at bookstores or call 505-899-3121. For this date you'll need to rent a nice hotel room. Call your mate from your room and have him or her come meet you there. When your partner arrives, be dressed in your robe, and have something sexy for your partner to slip into. Order strawberries (great for good breath) and champagne and celebrate your love.

23

♀ A Surprise Love Party—Throw your mate a surprise love party. Celebrate your love with a private bash.

24

♀ Friday Night Out—Remember when the two of you went on Friday or Saturday night dates? You couldn't wait to see each other! Put some of the magical time back into your relationship. Call your partner up and ask them if they'll go out with you next Friday night. Have them pack an overnighter bag & get dressed over a friend's house and pick them up from there.

25

♀ Mall Shopping Spree—Go to the mall and see what little goodies you can buy each other for $5.00 apiece. Gum, your favorite candy, a notepad, etc.

26

❧ Play the Dating Game—Both of you pick a number between 1 and 101. Go to the page in this book that particular numbered date is on. The two of you have to choose which date (pick the one that's either, the most reasonable, least expensive, most fun, etc.) you'll go on next week. The person who picks the date that loses implements the date both of you choose.

27

❧ Million Dollar Day—Spend the day together pretending you're millionaires. Test drive your dreams cars, visit expensive model homes in your area, go to fancy boutiques and pick out fantasy items you'd buy if you ever become millionaires. (You never know—you just might win the lottery!)

To love one who loves you, to admire one who

admires you, in a word, to be the idol of one's idol, is

exceeding the

limit of human joy;

it is stealing fire from heaven.

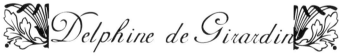

Delphine de Girardin

To love is to place our

happiness

in the happiness of another.

Gottfried Wilhem von Leibnitz

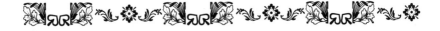

Love, she said, "seems to pump me full of vitamins. It makes me feel as if the sun were shining

and my hat was right

and my shoes were right and my frock was right and

my stockings were right, and somebody had just left

me *ten thousand a year*."

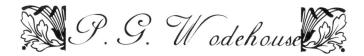

P. G. Wodehouse

Can't Buy Love

Romance doesn't have to be expensive. It just has to feel good. Here's a list of low-cost or free getaways:

28

Love In The Afternoon—Enjoy a private picnic together. Pack a picnic lunch with some inexpensive wine and a blanket in your car and head to a nice park or lake.

29

Sunday Driving—Take a drive in the country one Sunday afternoon. See if you can find a secluded place near a beautiful shade tree or babbling brook where the two of you can take a romantic walk or just enjoy the drive.

30

Seeing The Sights—Visit a local museum or art gallery together. Most museums charge an inexpensive entry fee.

31

Sweets For Your Sweet—Instead of going out to dinner, go out and just have dessert.

32

I Wanna Hold Your Hand—Take a romantic walk holding hands in the moonlight. (or in the afternoon, or early morning hours)

⌊33⌋

💲 Bringin' It On Home—Rent a couple of your favorite videos, pop some popcorn, curl up on the sofa, and watch them together. *500 Best American Films to Buy, Rent or Videotape*, by the editors of Films in Review, lists some of the all-time favorite videos.

⌊34⌋

💲 Sunlit Love—Get up early and watch the sunrise together.

⌊35⌋

💲 Breakfast In Bed—Take turns serving each other breakfast in bed. Invest in a breakfast tray and a silk, rose.

⌊36⌋

💲 Midnight Rendezvous—Serve up a delectable midnight rendezvous candlelight dinner for two. This one's great if you have little ones at home who like to stay up on the weekends. After they've gone to bed, the two of you can set your alarm for a romantic midnight meal.

Love is staying awake all

night with a sick child,

or a very healthy adult.

David Frost

ere are a man and a woman, being married. The entire world of summer lawns holds its breath for the event. The trees around them are lovely, displaying the small breath and motions of August. The couple glance at one another. Where has the moon gone, the requisite moon? Nearby, a mother begs her child, "Try to remember; when did you have it last?" Oh, impossible mystery. Where is joy when it is not here? Time says nothing. These things can happen, and will, while children at the yard's border play among grown-ups tasting the summer's wine.

David Keller, from "Afternoon, in a Back Yard on Chestnut Street"

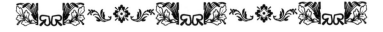

Married-With Children

Romance does not have to die after the children come along. In fact, your children can help you in your never-ending quest for romance. One of the best gifts you can give your children is a happy home life. That begins with the two of you being happy as a couple. By letting them see and share in the love you have for one another, you're setting an example for the way they'll act when they're married.

37

Mom & Dad = LOVE—Have your kids help you plan a surprise date with your partner. Let them help you pick the restaurant, pick out a gift or a card. Have them make up their own card they can give to both of you on your way out to celebrate.

38

House Swapping—Swap houses overnight with a neighbor, relative, or friend who does not have kids. They'll enjoy your kids for an evening, and you two will enjoy the privacy.

39

Sitter's Co-op—Form an informal sitting co-op with one or more friends who'll watch your kids when you go on romantic getaways, and you'll return the favor.

40

The Vacation Club—Instead of going on one vacation that lasts for two weeks, go on two vacations a year. One family vacation, and one romantic vacation. If you can't afford to go away to an expensive resort after you've spent a lot of money on a family vacation, go to a local hotel for a couple of days for your romantic getaway.

41

Visiting The Grandparents—Let your kids spend some time with their grandparents. While they're away, fill your days with romantic dates.

42

3 or 4 or maybe more—Go out on a "family date". Everyone gets dressed up & puts on the best behavior to go out to dinner. This one gives couples who have children a chance to show them how much fun mom & dad have when they go out. This is a good one for step-families. It's also an excellent one to show teens who are just beginning to date, what a good date is—unfortunately some teens are under the impression that a date is little more than necking in the back seat of a car.

43

Do Not Disturb—This is a great idea when you want some time alone as a couple—even if you have young children. Hang a do not disturb sign out on your bedroom door. If your children are too young to read—paint one side of the sign red or blue—tell them when the sign is hanging red (or blue) side out—it means—don't knock unless you're bleeding from head to toe. Of course for the little ones, it'll take awhile to reinforce them not knocking on the door, but you'll be pleasantly surprised—they'll get the hang of it sooner than you think!

Their correspondence was something like a

duet between a tuba and a piccolo.

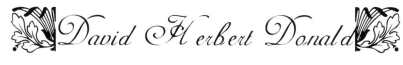

David Herbert Donald

(On love letters of Thomas Wolfe & Aline Bernstein)

At the touch of love everyone becomes a poet.

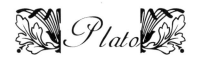

Plato

There is only one situation I can think of in

which men & women make an effort to read better

than they usually do. It is when they are in love and

reading a love letter.

Mortimer Adler

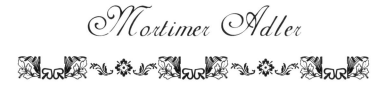

Love Means Never Having To Say You're Sorry.
(Not in this life)

If you're like most couples who've been together for awhile, that famous quote does not apply. Let's face it. In a perfect world, love may be so spiritually expressed that you always know when your partner is genuinely sorry when he or she hurts your feelings or does something that makes you feel let down. But in the real world of love & marriage and long-term commitment, most of us want to the I'm sorrys to be expressed verbally or at least by our partner's actions. There are also other things we'd like expressed from time to time. Which brings us to our next section...

Love Notes

44

Send a Card a Day—Send your mate a card a day for five days. In each card, tell them you can't wait for the special date you have planned for the fifth day. Say things like...

Can't wait for our special date...

It'll just be me & you...

Can't wait to hold you...

45

↙ Say it Out Loud—Take out an ad in your local paper asking your partner to go out on a special date with you. Put your office phone number in the ad and instruct your mate to call you to say yes or no. Make sure you circle the ad and leave it where your partner will be sure to find it.

46

↙ I'm Sorry—This one comes in handy when you've done something that you want to apologize for. Write a sincere note letting your partner know how you feel. Ask them to call you or meet with you after they've read the note so you can move into the making up stage.

47

↙ Lipstick Love—Write a note on the bathroom mirror with lipstick or soap that says: *I Love You! Will you be my date tonight?*

48

⚬ Long Distance Love—When you know you two are going to be separated by distance, buy some stationery and romantic cards and write each other. It's the perfect way to keep the home fires burning while you're away. When you do get back together, make sure to plan a special Welcome Home! celebration.

49

⚬ For Your Eyes Only—This is another one you can do when you're separated by distance. Write each other special "for your eyes only" love letters. Scent the letters with perfume or cologne and keep them in a special keepsake box. In the letters, tell your partner about a special fantasy date you'd like to have. When we were separated for an entire year because of Earl's job, Earl told me about a fantasy of being on a secluded island in the Bahamas. When we got back together, I surprised him with tickets for a 4-day cruise in Barbados.

50

⚬ Here, There & Everywhere—Leave little love notes for your mate...
In the car...
In his suit pocket...
In her purse...

Tacked on the mirror...

asking...

Do you want to fool around tonight?

How about a hot date tomorrow?

Would you like to have lunch with me?

You look so hot today! Will you be my date?

⟆51⟄

↪ You Deserve a Break—Write your partner the following note and leave it tacked on the refrigerator:

You deserve a break today! Don't bother cooking—I'm taking you out to dinner!

⟆52⟄

↪ Meet Me.♥.♥.—Leave a note your partner will find after coming home from work. In the note, ask your partner to meet you at your favorite lounge. One couple played out the fantasy of meeting each other at the lounge and pretending they didn't know each other. They sat at different tables and Dave had the bartender send Carol, (his wife) a drink and a note asking her if she'd join him. She did.

53

✎ Skywriting—Hire a skywriter to ask your mate on a date.

54

✎ Sending You My Love—Send your mate a telegram asking for the pleasure of his or her company.

55

✎ Sending You My Love Part Two—We all love to get (pleasant) surprises in the mail. Write a sexy love letter asking your mate for an evening out.

56

✎ Red, HOT Love—Get some matches from your favorite restaurant and write the following note, *"I'm hot for you! Meet me tonight for dinner at 7:00."*

Romantic Resources

Resources for writing romantic notes & love letters:

Love Letters: An Anthology of Passion, Michelle Lovric
Love's Witness, Jill Hollis
Wedding Readings, Eleanor Monroe

revity may be the soul of wit, but not when someone's saying "I love you." When someone's saying "I love you," he always ought to give a lot of details: Like, why does he love you? And, how much does he love you And when and here did he first begin to love you? Favorable comparisons with all other women he ever loved are also welcome. And even though he insists it would take forever to count the ways in which he loves you, let him start counting.

Judith Viorst

From The Telephone

Out of the dark cup

Your voice broke like a flower.

It trembled, swaying on its taut stem.

The caress in its touch

Made my eyes close.

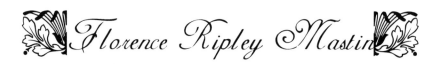
Florence Ripley Mastin

Phone Play

57

Just Called to Say I Love You—Call up your mate's job and leave a special message. Start the message with Stevie Wonder's *I Just Called To Say I Love You* playing (play it on a cassette or CD player). After it plays a while, break in and make a date for an extended coffee break during the week.

58

Reach Out & Touch—The phone is one of the best romantic devices you can have during any period of separation. Whenever job duties or anything separate the two of you, make sure you keep in romantic touch using the telephone. Make a "date" to call each other at a specified time every night.

⌊59⌋

❀ Call Your Spouse and Ask For a Date. Yes, even if you are married. Doing little things like this unexpectedly helps keep your marriage full of sizzle.

⌊60⌋

❀ I Love You, I LOVE YOU—Call your partner's answering machine on the job and leave an I love you message everyday for a week. Each day, plan a special rendezvous....

Day 1...Dinner by candlelight

Day 2...Take a bath together

Day 3...Watch your favorite romantic video together

Day 4...Take a walk in the moonlight holding hands

Day 5...Go up on the crest and watch the sparkle of the city lights together

Have everything prepared. Leave special instructions for your partner for each day.

Can there be any day but this?

Though many suns to shine endeavor?

We count three hundred, but we miss:

There is but one, and that one ever.

George Herbert, from "Easter"

Time is

Too slow for those who wait,
Too swift for those who fear,
Too long for those who grieve,
Too short for those who rejoice,
But for those who love, time is Eternity.
Hours fly, Flowers die,
New days, New ways, Pass by.
Love stays.

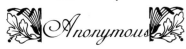

(inscription on a sundial at the University of Virginia)

Time Out For Love

61

Weekends are made for FUN—Hire a maid service that will come in and clean your house from top to bottom. Spend the time the two of you would have spent doing chores doing whatever you like. To find a reputable service in your area, look in the Yellow Pages under Maids' & Butlers' Service.

62

⏱   Take Time Off From Work—Take a week off from work and go to an exotic place for a romantic getaway for two.

63

⏱   Take a Special Lunch Break—Make a date to have a nice lunch with your partner. One man showed up on his wife's job with a picnic basket. They had a romantic lunch in her office.

64

⏱   Time Out From Cooking—Have a romantic dinner for two catered in.

65

⏱   Relax and Unwind—Make it an occasional dating habit to have a relaxing glass of wine together before dinner. Especially with two-income families in the rush-rush world, it's easy to come home from work and dive into your second job—taking care of home and family.

66

◷ Time Out for YOU—Buy your mate a gift certificate for a shopping spree or a special treatment in a beauty salon. While your mate is getting his or her special treat, use that time to do whatever it is you enjoy. People involved in long-term relationships understand that time out for self is just as important as time spent together.

If there is anything better than to be loved—it is loving.

Anonymous

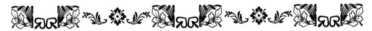

The only thing better than a chocolate ice cream

cone is sharing it with someone you love.

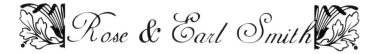

Rose & Earl Smith

Chocolate Love

Chocolate Trivia:

Is chocolate an aphrodisiac? Reliable sources tend to tell us it is:

• Chocolate contains large amounts of phenylethylamine, a chemical that is also produced by the body when one has amorous feelings.

• Some ancient civilizations thought chocolate was such a powerful arousal stimulant that the women were forbidden from having it.

• Debra Waterhouse's book, *Why Women Need Chocolate*, supports the feel-good theory. She encourages women to include limited amounts of chocolate in their diet.

67

🖋 Made With Love—Bake your mate a chocolate cake. Serve it for a special romantic dessert date.

68

🖋 A Chocolate Lover's Dream—While on a honeymoon getaway, visit a chocolate factory together. Here are some of the more famous ones:

Ethel M Chocolate Factory
2 Cactus Garden Dr.
Henderson, NV 89014
Free Tours Daily 8:30 a.m. - 5:30 p.m. Call 800-634-6584

Located 15 minutes from the Las Vegas Strip, the Ethel M Chocolate Factory is a delightful tour for chocolate lovers. An added bonus is their beautiful Cactus Garden, also part of the free tour.

In the heart of Hershey, Pennsylvania lies Chocolate World. You can go on the 15 minute tour of the factory, then visit the garden, wild-life park and amusement park.

Chocolate World
Box 800 Park Blvd.
Hershey, PA 17038

Call 717-534-4900

How about some Swiss chocolate? If you're ever in Europe, you can visit the Nestle chocolate factory.

Nestle
Service des Visites
1636 Broc FR
Switzerland (Phone)(41) 296-5151—Call or write for reservations.

⌐69⌐

⚓ Chocolate Chip Love—Bake your partner some chocolate chip cookies for lunch one day during the week. Wrap the cookies in plastic and attach a note to the cookies that says: *This is just a small sample of goodies I've got in store for you—We've got a hot date tonight. Meet me at 7:05.*

70

We LIVE For Chocolate—Go on a chocolate shopping spree. Go to your favorite candy store or ice cream parlor and enjoy your favorite chocolate treat together.

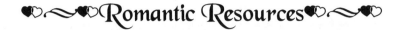 Romantic Resources

Catalogs for Chocolate Lovers

Hershey's...717-534-4200
Celebration Fantastic
(This great company features chocolate gifts & more for special occasions, they also offer chocolate-stemmed roses in their Valentine's Day catalog).......................................800-527-6566
Lyla's Chocolates...415-383-8887
(This company has a wonderful array of chocolates including the Golden Gate Bridge, chocolate-stemmed roses and more)

Love is a spiritual fire.

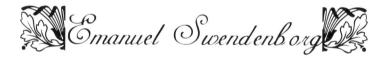

Emanuel Swendenborg

You glow in my heart
Like the flames of uncounted candles.

Amy Lowell

Soft Lights & Candlelight

⌣71⌣

🕯 Turn the Lights Down Low—Make a slow and easy date that starts and ends in your bedroom. Get some soft lights—mood lights for your bedroom, put on Smokey Robinson's sexy song, *Baby, Come Close*, or Teddy Pendegrass's, *Turn Out The Lights*, on your cassette or CD player. Relax and enjoy each other's company.

⌣72⌣

🕯 Do Not Disturb—Turn your bedroom into a hotel room! Light some candles, serve up some drinks on a dining tray or cart, and hang out a do-not-disturb sign on your bedroom door. You'll be surprised at how doing a little thing like imagining the two of you are escaping from your familiar surroundings will do to put some zest back into your love life!

73

§ Viva La' LOVE! One man from Toledo, Ohio got very creative with this candlelight idea. When he found out his wife's dream was to visit romantic Paris, France, he set-up his backyard like an outdoor Paris cafe. He had the table dressed in a red and white checkered tablecloth, with French bread and wine. Then, he lit 100 candles he had placed all over the backyard. Dressed like a French waiter, beret and all—he served his wife dinner on a covered silver platter. When she took the cover off the platter, she found two round trip tickets to Paris.

74

§ Make Love by Candlelight—Turn ordinary lovemaking into something special by lighting scented candles and making love by the iridescent light of the candles.

Love does not consist in gazing at each other

but in looking outward together in the same direction.

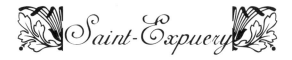

Saint-Expuery

I just want you to love me,

primal doubts and all.

William Holden

(as Max Schumacher in *Network*)

Movie Mania

75

Vintage Movies—Go to a vintage movie house together. Vintage movie houses often run old movies guaranteed to spark romance.

76

Movie Marathon—Have a movie marathon in your home. Rent or buy a bunch of videos and watch 3, 4, or 5 of them. This date is one that can last all night!

77

Steamy Love—Go to a drive-in movie together. Your main purpose? To steam up those car windows!

78

Remember When—Rent a couple of videos that take you back to when the two of you were dating. Curl up on the sofa, enjoy the movies and reminiscence.

79

Movie Trivia—Play a movie trivia game together. Pick a movie (on video) you've both seen before & both enjoyed. Watch the movie one night and pick out little trivia questions you can ask each other about the movie. Example, what is the star carrying when he locks his keys in the car? Put the movie aside (with the questions tucked inside the video jacket) for awhile. When you watch the movie again, play the game. Make fun bets with each other, like loser serves winner breakfast in bed.

80

Stars In The Family—Make an annual date to watch a fun or romantic video starring the two of you. One couple from New York watch their wedding video on every anniversary. They say it makes brings back wonderful memories and makes them want to get married all over again. They plan on renewing their vows on their twentieth wedding anniversary.

Romantic Resources

Video picks for movie lovers:

Here are some video suggestions first by category followed by a list a the 50 top grossing movies of all time.

Adventure:

The Adventures of Robin Hood
Jaws
King Kong
Lost Horizon
The Maltese Falcon
Raiders of the Lost Ark
20,000 Leagues Under the Sea
The Long Voyage Home
David Copperfield
Bonnie & Clyde

Sci-fi/Fantasy

Terminator
Superman
Total Recall
The Picture of Dorian Gray
Planet of the Apes
Poltergeist
The 7th Voyage of Sinbad
Star Wars
The Wizard of Oz
WarGames

Drama

All the President's Men
Bang the Drum Slowly

Cool Hand Luke
Coal Miner's Daughter
The Godfather
From Here to Eternity
Midnight Cowboy
Sophie's Choice
12 Angry Men
To Kill a Mockingbird

Musical

An American in Paris
Cabaret
Funny Face
The Great Ziegfeld
Jailhouse Rock
Mary Poppins
The Music Man
Oklahoma!

The Rose
That's Entertainment!

Romantic Classics

The African Queen
Gone With the Wind
The Best Years of Our Lives
Wuthering Heights
Heaven Can Wait
A Star is Born
My Fair Lady
Splendor in the Grass
Seven Brides For Seven Brothers
Love Me Tonight

African-American Romance Classics

Carmen Jones

Nothing But A Man
For Love of Ivy
Sounder
Claudine
Coming to America
Paris Blues
Lady Sings the Blues
Mahogany
A Warm December

Western

The Magnificent Seven
The Professionals
She Wore a Yellow Ribbon
Unforgiven
True Grit
Red River
Shane
The Wild Bunch
Winchester 73
Wili Penny

Modern Love Stories

The Bodyguard
Dances With Wolves
Beauty & the Beast
Bram Stoker's Dracula
Pretty Woman
Ghost
Robin Hood: Prince of Thieves
Sleepless in Seattle
Scent of a Woman
Jason's Lyric

All-Time Top 50 American Movies

1. Jurassic Park
2. E.T.
3. Star Wars
4. Return of the Jedi
5. Batman

6. The Empire Strikes Back
7. Home Alone
8. Ghostbusters
9. Jaws
10. Raiders of the Lost Ark
11. Indiana Jones & the Last Crusade
12. Terminator 2
13. Indiana Jones & the Temple of Doom
14. Beverly Hills Cop
15. Back to the Future
16. Home Alone 2
17. Batman Returns
18. Ghost
19. Grease
20. Tootsie
21. The Exorcist
22. Rain Man
23. The Godfather
24. Robin Hood: Prince of Thieves
24. Superman
25. Close Encounters of the Third Kind
27. Pretty Woman
28. Dances with Wolves
29. Three Men & a Baby
30. Who Framed Roger Rabbit
31. Beverly Hills Cop II
32. Lethal Weapon 3
33. The Sound of Music
34. Gremlins
35. Lethal Weapon 2
36. Top Gun
37. Gone With the Wind
38. Rambo: First Blood Part II
39. The Sting
40. Rocky IV
41. Saturday Night Fever
42. Back to the Future, Part II

43. Honey, I Shrunk the Kids
44. National Lampoon's
    Animal House
45. Crocodile Dundee
46. Fatal Attraction
47. Platoon
48. Beauty and the Beast
49. Look Who's Talking
50. 101 Dalmatians

There are three sights which warm my heart and are beautiful in the eyes of the Lord and of men: concord among brothers, friendship among neighbors, and a man & wife who are inseparable.

from The Wisdom of Ben Sira, Chapter 25, Verse I

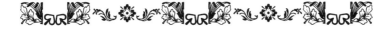

simple enough pleasure surely to have breakfast alone with one's husband, but how seldom married people in the midst of life achieve it.

Anne Morrow Lindbergh

Silk, Satin & Lace

Few things heat things up in the bedroom as quickly as sexy underwear. Here are some dates centered around sexy lingerie and silky boxer shorts.

81

The Grab Bag—This one's fun especially if you're in the rut of wearing the same 'not tonight I have a headache' garb to bed every night. Put some lingerie & boxer shorts in a shopping size bag. Have your partner pick an outfit for you and you pick one for your partner. Enjoy an unforgettable evening under the sheets.

82

🖊 Go On Location—Get dressed up in beautiful peignoir & meet your partner on location, on the couch, in front of the fireplace, or in another bedroom in the house. Keep the lighting low for a sultry effect.

83

🖊 For Your Eyes Only—Have a For your eyes only fashion show. Send your partner a ticket that reads, *Tonight's the night*! You can even cut the invitation out in the form of some sexy briefs.

84

🖊 Let's Go Shopping!—Make a date to go shopping for lingerie & undergarments. Buy something you'd like to see your partner in and have your partner buy something for you.

85

Ordering In—Have a shop at home day for lingerie. Together browse through some sexy lingerie & swimwear catalogs.

86

Have a Lingerie Party—Invite a group of friends (couples) over and have a home lingerie fashion show. An outfit called Undercoverwear is the largest supplier for these home fashion shows. They will have a trained fashion consultant come into your home and show their latest line of underdress. In the couple parties, each couple gets their turn to go into a private room or bathroom to try on things they'd like to buy for each other. To find out more about these fun fashion shows you can call Undercoverwear at 617-938-0007 or Lotions & Lace at 702-796-9966 .

87

Reading is Fun—Buy a romance novel and read excerpts to each other. Be sure to dress for the occasion. (dress sexy)

I like to laugh and be happy

With a beautiful kiss,

I tell you, in all the world

There is no bliss like this.

Stevie Smith

What is a kiss?

Why this as some approve:

The sure, sweet cement, glue,

and lime of love.

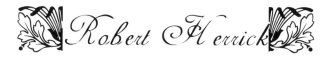 Robert Herrick

Kissing Couples

 little Kissing Trivia:

Kissing keeps wrinkles away. A passionate smacker uses 29 facial muscles. (It's the kind of exercise that feels good, too)

Kissing helps alleviate stress. Sex & kissing both release that Dr. Feelgood chemical, phenylethylamine (also found in chocolate.)

Kissing is the world's best (and most overlooked) natural aphrodisiac.

⌊88⌋

❈ Sometimes It's Better In The Back Seat—Go for a night time drive and find a secluded place. Neck in the back seat of your car.

⌊89⌋

❈ New Kinds Of Kisses—*The Art of Kissing*, by William Cane has several different kinds of fun kisses. Reserve some time one afternoon and go through the book and pick out your favorites. Here's a sample:

> ❈The Vacuum Kiss   ❈The Music Kiss
> ❈The French Kiss   ❈The Candy Kiss
> ❈The Perfume Kiss   ❈The Surprise Kiss

Try your favorites and make up some of your own.

⌊90⌋

❈ Kiss-n-Tell—This one's fun. Have a professional necking session. Make-out with your partner—just kissing—no sex. After a few minutes (or more) of making out, each of you tell the other what you loved about the making out session. Focus only on the positive. This is a great one for reinforcing what you like about how your partner holds you, kisses you, etc. and vice-versa.

91

❈ Kissin' & Fishin'—This one comes from a couple who live in Toledo, Ohio. Since they both enjoy bass fishing, Bob bought his wife, Sue, a new fishing pole. They went bass fishing and he didn't even get mad when she caught more fish than he did, because they played a game of kissing after each catch. (Wouldn't you say this couple knows a thing or two about reeling them in?)

92

❈ Honey, I'm Home—Ever have trouble getting your partner to listen to you when come home from work? Try this: Instead of usual peck on the cheek, grab your lover and give him or her a long, lusty smooch. Tell them how much you missed them today. Then spend five or ten minutes telling your partner what went on in your day. (We're sure you'll have your partner's attention.)

93

❈ The 10-second Kiss—How long does your usual kiss last? If you're like most couples, a peck on the cheek takes a millisecond. Try the ten second kiss on for size. Be sure to time it at first, so you'll see the difference. After awhile, kissing and holding each other longer will become routine.

Romantic Resources

More Kissing Trivia:

Memorable Kisses (From The Book of Lists)

The Kiss of Life

It was a kiss from God that infused the spirit of life into man, according to the account of Genesis (2:7). God is said to have formed Adam from slime and dust and then breathed a rational soul into him.

The Kiss in Iberian Stone (c. 300–100 BC)

One the earliest depiction's of a kiss between a man and woman is on an Iberian stone relief dating from the 4th to the 2nd century BC. The piece, featuring the kissers in profile from the shoulders up, was found in Osuna, Spain, and is currently on exhibit in the Madrid National Archeological Museum.

The Kiss That Cost Thomas Saverland His Nose

In 1837, at the dawn of the Victorian Era in Great Britain, Thomas Saverland attempted to kiss Caroline Newton in a light–hearted manner. Rejecting Saverland's pass, Miss Newton not so lightheartedly bit off part of his nose. Saverland took Newton to court, but she was acquitted. "When a man kisses a woman against her will," ruled the judge, "she is fully entitled to bite his nose, if she so pleases." "And eat it up," added a barrister.

The Kiss by Francois Auguste Rodin (1886)

One of the most renowned pieces of sculpture in the Western world is The Kiss, sculpted by French artist Francois Auguste Rodin in 1886. Inspired by Dante, the figure of two nude lovers kissing brought the era of classical art to an end. Rodin described The Kiss as "complete in itself and artificially set apart from the surrounding world."

The First Kiss Recorded on Film (1896)

The first kiss ever to be recorded in a motion picture occurred in Thomas Edison's film The Kiss between John C. Rice and actress May Irwin in April, 1896. Adapted from a short scene in the Broadway comedy The Widow Jones, The Kiss was filmed by Raff and Gammon for nickelodeon audiences. Its running time was less than 30 seconds.

The Most Often Kissed Statue in History (late 1800's)

The figure of Guidarello Guidarelli, a fearless 16th—century Italian soldier, was sculpted in marble by Tullio Lombardo (c. 1455—1532) and put on display at the Academy of Fine Arts in Ravenna, Italy. During the late 1800s, a rumor started that any woman who kissed the reclining, armor—clad statue would marry a wonderful gentleman and settle down with him. Some four to five million superstitious women have since kissed Guidarelli's cold marble lips. Consequently, the soldier's mouth has acquired a faint reddish glow.

The Movie with 191 Kisses

In 1926 Warner Brothers Studios starred John Barrymore in Don Juan. During the course of the film (2 hr. 47 min.), the amorous adventurer bestows a total of 191 kisses on a number of beautiful señoritas—an average of one every 53 seconds.

The Longest Kiss on Film

The longest kiss in motion picture history is between Jane Wyman and Regis Toomey in the 1941 production of You're in the Army Now. The Lewis Seiler comedy about two vacuum cleaner salesmen features a scene in which Toomey and Wyman hold a single kiss for 3 minutes and 5 seconds.

The Kiss That Cost $1,260 (1977)

Ruth van Herpen visited an art museum in Oxford, England, in 1977 and kissed a painting by American artist Jo Baer, leaving red lipstick stains on the $18,000 work. Restoration costs were reported to be as much as $1,260. Appearing in court, van Herpen explained, "I only kissed it to cheer it up. It looked so cold."

The Longest Kiss on Record

The longest kiss in a "smoochathon" was held between Bobbi Sherlock and Ray Blazina in Pittsburgh, Pa., between May 1 and 6, 1978. Their record lasted 130 hr. 2 min. (A smoochothan sounds like a great idea for you and your mate! Only, in your smoochathon, make a day long event where you kiss every time you enter the same room.)

You are my { husband/wife }

My feet shall run because of you.

My feet, dance because of you.

My heart shall beat because of you.

My eyes, see because of you.

My mind, think because of you

And I shall love because of you.

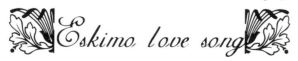 Eskimo love song

We discovered in each other and ourselves worlds, galaxies, a universe.

Anne Rivers Siddons

Reservations For Two

94

The Honeymooners—One of the best dates you can have with your mate is one you both should resolve to do annually. Make plans every year to go on a Honeymoon Getaway. It can be done on your anniversary, if convenient, or anytime during the year it's convenient for the two of you to make the great, honeymoon escape. There's a physiological reason you call these honeymoon getaways, not anniversary getaways. The honeymoon is always seen as the romantic time in marriage that fades too quickly. By going on a honeymoon getaway, you're making a point to recreate this ambiance every year.

Thus you have a never-ending honeymoon. When you make your escape, it can be as elaborate as going to the Caribbean on a secluded island, or as inexpensive as renting a local hotel room for an overnighter. It doesn't matter how long you get away, only that you go somewhere every year to relive your honeymoon. This one date alone is guaranteed to work wonders for your intimate relationship.

95

Cruisin'—Go on a romantic cruise getaway. Cruise to an exotic port, drink in the sights together, and enjoy a few days, or weeks of romantic bliss. Listed in the Resource Section are numbers of cruise ships and discount travel clubs.

96

Join A Vacation Club—One of the best ways to guarantee a quality vacation for the two of you every year is to join a Vacation Club. With a Vacation Club, you purchase a week (or more) at a specified resort. You can travel to that resort during a specified time every year, or you can trade your week for a week at another resort in an exotic place. And unlike hotels, most of these resorts come furnished with kitchenware & kitchens, some have VCR's and other amenities in the rooms. It's a great way to make your annual escapes at bargain rates. Here are the names of some Vacation Clubs:

Sedona Vacation Club/Los Abrigados   (Sedona, AR)(This is a beautiful resort) 602-282-1777
Club Florida Villas (Orlando, FL) 1-800-373-8455

97

A Hole-In One—Can't afford an expensive trip? Don't worry—you can create your own paradise. One woman took this suggestion to a new level. She and her husband both love to golf. So while he was away golfing in an out-of-town tournament, she surprised him by arranging to have dessert and wine served to them—on the hometown golf course. Upon his return, he was instructed to meet her at the golf course at dusk. She was there waiting for him with their waiter who served them their delicious dessert at their own private table seated in the middle of the course. She had made arrangements for all of this with the golf course manager. She said she and her husband and their special date are still the talk of the town!

98

❈ Breakfast In Bed—Plan a special getaway at a local bed & breakfast. Here's what one couple wrote in their diary after returning from their getaway date:

Lost: one load of stress & fatigue...
somewhere between the hot tub,
under the stars,
and the cool sheets of a perfect bed.
If found please do not return it to us,
nor take it on yourselves,
but go to your favorite hideaway
& let it get lost again.

Reputable bed & breakfast inns offer a unique romantic experience.

99

❈ My Mind Escapes Me—This date takes you away in a sense—only it's an escape in your mind. This idea comes from a couple that say they keep the homes fires burning bright by playing out a little fantasy they call: I've been watching you. Every now and then, Kim will call Steve on his job and say something like, "You don't know me, but I've seen you around town, and I think you're really hot." She'll play this scenario out for about a week or so, calling him up and telling him what she loves about him. She tops the fantasy off by finally saying, "Can we meet somewhere in secret?" They swear that after playing that scenario out and meeting in their secret place, the fireworks fly for weeks afterwards. Steve also plays the role of the pursuer from time to time.

⌣100⌣

More Mind Games—Another variation of this mind-game comes from a disc jockey in Minneapolis. He made a date with his wife, where he picked her up at a friend's house, just like they did before they got married. But when he rang the doorbell, he said she was shocked when she opened the door and found him dressed in black leather from head to toe with his hair slicked back. For the entire night, he actually became an alter-ego, talking, walking, and looking different from his usual self. They both had a great time and when they went home he says, "We made love like rabbits."

⌣101⌣

Under The Stars—Go on a camping trip together. You'll be surprised at how gazing at a little star-light in the beautiful outdoors can spark your romance.

⌣102⌣

🮲 Once In A Lifetime—Every now & then, for special occasions, or just because, do the out-of-the-ordinary-once-in-a-lifetime-date. Rent a limo and go to a top-notch restaurant Or, go on a once in a lifetime wildly expensive, wildly romantic & wildly exotic vacation. One of the best we've heard about is offered by an outfit called Villas of the World, where you can rent a 15,000 square foot mansion on a secluded Island in the Caribbean with 24 hour limousine service and a maid & butler staff of six. The cost? $15,000 & up for one week. Villas of the World has other, more reasonable holiday getaways. Call them at 1-800-222-6235 for more information. See the Romantic Resource Section for more once in a lifetime getaways.

❤.~❤Romantic Resources❤.~❤

Cruise Information:

Carnival 800-327-7276
Norwegian Cruise Line 800-832-1122
Royal Viking Cruises 800-426-0821
Windjammer Barefoot Cruises.. 800-327-2601
Windstar Sail Cruises 800-258-7245
Princess Cruise Line 800-LOVEBOAT

For Savings

Check out cruise rates from the following:
South Florida Cruise 800-327-SHIP
(Say they can save you 5 to 50% on brochure rates)
PriceCostco Travel—PriceCostco offers substantial travel discounts on cruises and other travels to it's members. For more information, call PriceCostco Travel at 1-800-800-8505.

The Cruise Line 800-777-0707 (They publish a free magazine three times a year with updates on cruises and special deals on specific trips.)

Bed & Breakfast Info:

Bed & Breakfast USA 914-271-6228
Croton-On-Hudson
New York, NY 10521

Bed & Breakfast International 415-525-4569
151 Ardmore Rd.
Kesington, CA 94707

More Bomantic Getaways

Alaska—Tauck Tours offers a thirteen-day experience that includes breakfast at the famous Space Needle Restaurant in Seattle, gold-mining at the Little Eldorado Gold Camp in Fairbanks, a ride on the sternwheel riverboat Discovery, a visit to Mount McKinley, a three-hour float-plane trip over some of the most spectacular scenery in North America, visits to Anchorage and Juneau, and a cruise through Glacier Bay on the way back to Vancouver and Seattle. Call 203-226-6911 for more information.

Hawaii—Classic Hawaii Custom Vacations can help you plan a romantic getaway for two at any of over one hundred properties on six different islands (Hawaii, Kauai, Lanai, Maui, Molokai, and Oahu). Call 800-221-3949 for more information.

Club Med—Club Med offers escapes for couples to such romantic places as French Polynesia, the Caribbean, and the Bahamas. At a Club Med, couples can spend their days relaxing alone or can choose from a wonderful list of his-and-hers activities, including swimming, scuba diving, water skiing, sailing, wind surfing, snorkeling, golf, and tennis. Call 800-258-2633 for more information.

Europe—A vacation in Europe, arranged by a company called Cosmos Tourama, offers some of the best values available. They manage over fifty tours ranging in length from eight days to a month, the decision is yours, based on the tour you choose. Call 800-888-7292 for more information.

Love

is the heart's immortal thirst

to be completely known

and all forgiven.

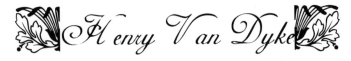

Henry Van Dyke

They gave each other a smile with a future in it.

Ring Lardner

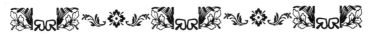

A Few More for the Road

Similar to Lay's potato chips, we just couldn't stop at 101. We received so many creative dating ideas from couples around the country, we've included a bonus section of dates in potpourri form.

One of the most common mistakes couples in long-term relationships make is thinking that at some point in their relationship, they 'outgrow' dating. A relationship is never to old to make dating merely a fond memory. Most people involved in a dateless relationship are too firmly planted in boring comfort with their relationship. By referring to this book often and using the creative dating ideas—you'll always find ways to keep your relationship 'forever young.'

103

❥More Chocolate Love—Share a bag of *M&Ms*. Did you know the green ones are aphrodisiacs? Feed the green ones to each other.
Here are some other ideas of chocolate lover's can share together:

● A box of chocolates—buy the kind Forest Gump recommends—the delectable ones where you never know what you're going to get.

● Fudge: Homemade fudge is delicious as well as store-bought fudge.

● Chocolate Cake or cupcakes: Bake a heart-shaped cake together.

● Chocolate Malt: Share one together on a Sunday afternoon.

104

❥Sharing Your Love—Brighten the day of someone in a nursing home by visiting them together. One of the most poetic things you can do in life is listen to someone who's loved a lifetime's worth talk about the partner who has died and left them behind. That person won't waste time talking about the deceased spouse's faults or shortcomings. He or she will talk instead about what matters most in the end—that they shared a wonderful life with someone special. This experience will make you count your blessings.

105

❤Drinks a la elegance—One radio DJ in Arizona says he and his wife make a date of visiting an elegant hotel lounge in the area for drinks. The hotel lobbies are usually very elaborate and many of them have fireplaces. This is a fun and inexpensive way to cozy up in a relaxed atmosphere.

106

❤Ringing in the New Year—Ring the New Year by having a romantic New Year's Eve party for two. Dress up, put on some of your favorite music and dance the night away. Make a special romantic toast to ring in the new year.

⌞107⌟

❤Kissing Me Softly—Go for a drive and kiss during the red lights. Here are some other kissing ideas:

Kiss each other from head-to-toe.

Kiss everytime you see your dream car on the road.

Sneak into a private corner in a very public place (like a mall) & steal a kiss.

Go to a pediatric ward in a hospital and wave and throw kisses to all the babies.

⌞108⌟

❤Mother's Day—Celebrate Mother's Day by taking your moms out to lunch together. This one is great to do when you are just getting to know each other and you'd like to introduce your mothers to each other. One couple we know broke the news of their engagement to both of their mothers on Mother's Day when they took them out to lunch. Both mothers were deeply touched.

⌞109⌟

❤Halloween Romance—Dress up as a famous romantic couple (Romeo & Juliet—Bonnie & Clyde—Samson & Delilah) for Halloween. Go to a

Halloween bash in costume or just dress up for each other. Or, take your kids trick or treating, or if you don't have kids, go with friends who do, or play double-dare and go by yourselves. The person's who's bold enough to go to the door in costume asking for treats from your neighbors, wins the double-dare.

110

❤Welcome Home—Meet your mate at the airport after a trip. Greet him or her with a welcome home sign. You can even dress in something sexy and put on an overcoat to where inside the airport. When the two of you are alone, give your partner a preview of what's in store for him or her tonight!

111

❤Playing Around—Go to a putt-putt range and play golf together. This is a fun and relaxing way to get in a little exercise and do something different together.

112

❤Me, you & Oreos, too—Share some Oreo cookies together as an after dinner snack. Another cookie idea—spend the evening baking cookies together.

113

❤A Fax full of Love—Write a love note to your partner asking for a date. Fax it to your partner's computer.

114

❤More C O M P U T E R Love—Send each other sexy E-mail. Ask your mate for a date and send it E-mail. Have him or her respond by E-mail only.

115

❤Flower Power—Extend the life of roses you give your mate. When the roses are beginning to wither, throw them onto your bed and make love on the petals.

116

❤Paper Plate Love—Write a sexy love message on a paper plate and share it with your mate during mealtime.

117

❤Start a Romance Scrapbook—Spend some time going through old pictures of the two of you on dates or having fun together. Gather cards and letters you've written one another, etc. If you don't have any momentos, start saving some. Years from now you will cherish these momentos more than you know.

118

❤Meet me at the Airport—Meet at an airport bistro and have dinner one night. You can even get all dressed up and pretend you're flying away to a romantic getaway.

119

❤More Airport Romance—Spend an afternoon at the airport watching the planes take off and land. Make plans for your next romantic getaway. Sock away money from every paycheck to save for your getaway. Call it your couplefund.

⟟120⟍

❥Christmas Loving—Stay up at Christmas and make cookies for Santa. Make sure there's plenty of mistletoe hanging around.

⟟121⟍

❥It's a Celebration!—Instead of just celebrating your wedding anniversaries, make it a point to celebrate your dating anniversaries also.

⟟122⟍

❥Remember When—Spend an afternoon reminiscing about special dates you've shared in the past. See who has the best memory.

⟟123⟍

❥Memories—Start a dating journal. Record special memories of the dates you share. Make it a habit to record moments of dates you have together, special vacations you share, and how happy you make each other feel. One couple started a couple journal when they got married. They often write letters to one another in the journal.

⌊124⌋

❤Head 'Em Up–Move 'Em Out–Make a date out of an afternoon at the rodeo. Enjoy the western sights and atmosphere.

⌊125⌋

❤Hold a Clint Eastwood Marathon–Rent some of Clint Eastwood's old western & cop movies and watch them together. See who can do the best Eastwood (Make my day) imitation.   You can also hold marathons of other stars like John Wayne, Humphrey Bogart, Marilyn Monroe, Judy Garland, Sidney Poiter, etc.

⌊126⌋

❤Go on a D^3 Date–Go out for drinks, dinner, & dancing.

⌊127⌋

❤And the Award Goes to–Make a date of the Emmy's, Grammy's or Academy Awards. See who can pick the most winners. Winner gets to pick a date out of this book that his or her partner must carry out within a week. (There aren't any losers in this game.)

128

♥A Lying Next to You—Spend a rainy afternoon napping wrapped in each other's arms. Listen to the comforting sounds of the rainstorm.

129

♥A Special Weekend Date for Two—Meet at a tavern on a Saturday for lunch. This is a great one to do if both of you want to spend the morning running errands or doing something alone. After the alone-time, the two of you can meet at a local tavern and enjoy lunch together.

130

♥A Caroling We Go—Make a date to go Christmas caroling together. Bake some special goodies, take them to a retirement home and share songs, love & laughter. Both you and the senior citizens at the home will cherish the memories.

131

❤A Slumber Party—Enjoy a slumber party together. Spread some sleeping bags or blankets out on the living room floor, watch TV, pop popcorn, and spend the night staying up having fun.

132

❤Cool Love—Sneak wine coolers into a movie theater together. If you don't drink—sneak in something else like a candy-bar to share, some sodas or even some homemade popcorn.

133

❤A Sports Date—Buy tickets to see the Harlem Globetrotters. Another sports date can be trying on a new sport. Buy tickets to a sport the two of you have never watched before. Learn about it together.

134

❤Wake Me Up Early on Saturday—Get up early and watch Saturday morning cartoons together. Share a box of doughnuts.

⟍135⟋

❤Let's Go to the Zoo—Spend an afternoon together at the Zoo. Afterwards, talk about your favorite animals.

⟍136⟋

❤Model Love—Spend an afternoon putting together a toy model or flying a kite or a model airplane.

⟍137⟋

❤Let's Race—Make a date of driving around in carnival bumper cars or go-carts.

Another variation of enjoying yourselves at an amusement park: Visit Disneyland or DisneyWorld as honeymooners. It's one of the most romantic places for lovers.

⟍138⟋

❤Frostbitten by Love—Dress in warm clothing & go to a park or frozen pond and share a thermos of hot chocolate. Be sure to cuddle-up and keep each other warm.

139

❤Ooh baby, It's cold outside—Make a date of frolicking in the snow. Make a snowman, have a snowball fight, make snow angels. After freezing, cuddle up to a cozy fire in your fireplace and drink some hot apple cider.

140

❤Comedy Night Out—Go to a local club and catch a comedy act. Laughter feels great and it always helps love blossom when two lovers are in a good mood.

141

❤Out in the Woods—Have fun exploring an unknown path in the woods together or take up a new sport—hiking together. Make sure you don't venture too far off the beaten path so you don't get lost.

142

❤Let's strike it rich—Spend the day trying to win some cash. Play bingo, play the slots at a casino, and top it off by buying a lotto ticket together. Talk about how the two of you would spend the millions if you won.

143

❥Get Lost—Go on a drive during the weekend and get lost on purpose. See what adventures you can find to explore.

144

❥Down Memory Lane—Drive to your old neighborhood together. Better yet, rent an expensive sports car and drive past your old neighbors houses. Drop in to say hi.

145

❥Massage Me—Wash each other's hair and massage each other's scalp and brush each other's hair.

146

❥What If—Spend the afternoon playing what if. Share your deepest dreams and fantasies. Let yourself go and indulge in your wildest, most romantic, most expensive & most delectable dreams.

147

❤️Fingers Full of Love—Finger food can be very romantic. Have fun finger painting with chocolate pudding.

148

❤️A Finger Food Feast—Have fun having a finger food feast. Gather up your favorite finger foods—cake, pudding, cookies, candy, and take turns feeding each other. Add to the fun by having an innocent food fight!

149

❤️Me, You & Our Harley too—Rent a motorcycle, get dressed in black leather and explore the countryside together.

150

❤️ For Animal Lovers—Visit a pet shop together and make some new friends.

⌊151⌋

❤ Start a Ritual–Go to church together on Sundays, read the paper together, watch your favorite TV show together every week. Start a ritual date that will provide enjoyment and couple time together every week.

⌊152⌋

❤Celebrate 'I'm glad we Met'–Make a special date to celebrate the best part of your love–*The Day You Met*.

Through their kisses and caresses they experienced a joy and wonder the equal of which has never been known or heard of. But I shall be silent on this subject, for it should never be recounted; for the rarest and most delectable pleasures are those which are hinted at, but never told.

From Lancelot II, *Chretien de Troyes*

..he began to adore the hairs; a hundred thousand times he touched them to his eyes, his mouth, his forehead, and his cheeks. His joy was made manifest in every way, and he thought himself rich and happy indeed. He placed the hairs in his breast, close to his heart, between the shirt and the skin. He would not exchange them for a cartload of emeralds and carbuncles..

From the Book of Courtly Love
A knight admiring his lady-in-waiting

The Rules of Love Book I

From *De Arte Honesti Amandi* by Andreas Capellanus

In twelfth century France, knights who courted their ladies-in-waiting were called troubadours. They developed the art of courting and even had a highly elaborate, sophisticated, and aristocratic code of behavior. Theirs was a passionate code, and it still has a great influence on our culture and society, and the way we think about romance. We were pleasantly surprised to find that though a few of the rules of love are outdated, most of them hold true today because they're based on love, honor & respect for your partner.

1. Flee from avarice like a noxious plague, and embrace its opposite.

2. You must keep yourself chaste for your beloved's sake.

3. You must not deliberately try to break up a love affair between a woman suitably joined to another man.

4. Take care not to chose for your love a person whom a natural sense of shame would prohibit you from marrying.

5. At all costs take care to avoid lies.

6. Do not have many people in the secret of your love.

7. Being obedient in all things to the commands of ladies, always study to be enrolled in the service of love.

8. When fulfilling and recieving the pleasures of love, always let modesty be present.

9. Speak no evil.

10. Never publicly expose lovers.

11. Show yourself in all things polite and courteous.

12. When you are engaging in the pleasures of love, do not exceed the desires of your lover.

The Rules of Love Book II

From *De Arte Honesti Amandi* by Andreas Capellanus

1. The state of marriage does not properly excuse anyone from loving.

2. He who does not feel jealous is not capable of loving.

3. No one can love two people at the same time.

4. It is well-known that love is always either growing or declining.

5. Whatever a lover takes against his lover's will has no savor.

6. A male does not fall in love until he has reached full manhood.

7. A mourning period of two years for a deceased is required of the surviving partner.

8. No one should be prevented of loving except by reason of his own death.

9. No one can love unless they are compelled by the eloquence of love.

10. Love is accustomed to be an exile from the house of avarice.

11. It is unseemly to love anyone whom you would be ashamed to marry.

12. A true lover does not desire the passionate embraces of anyone else but his beloved.

13. Love that is made public rarely lasts.

14. Love easily obtained is of little value; difficulty in obtaining it makes it precious.

15. Every lover regularly turns pale in the presence of his beloved.

16. On suddenly catching sight of his beloved, the heart of a lover begins to palpitate.

17. A new love drives out the old.

18. A good character alone makes someone worthy of love.

19. If love lessens, it soon fails and rarely recovers.

20. A man in love is always fearful.

21. The feeling of love is always increased by true jealousy.

22. When a lover feels suspicious of his beloved, jealousy, and with it the sensation of love, are increased.

23. A man tormented by the thought of love eats and sleeps very little.

24. Everything a lover does ends in the thought of his beloved.

25. A true lover considers nothing good but what he thinks will please his beloved.

26. Love can deny nothing to love.

27. A lover cannot have too much of his beloved's consolations.

28. A small supposition compels a lover to suspect his beloved of doing wrong.

29. A man who is troubled by excessive lust does not usually love.

30. A true lover is continually and without interruption obsessed by the image of his beloved.

31. Nothing forbids one woman being loved by two men, or one man by two women.

One word of advice:
For those of you poised to go out and plan the most romantic date of a lifetime, make sure to get your partner's input before putting undue time and effort into a date that's not up your spouse's alley. Find out what your partner considers romantic. If he or she can't get enough of the outdoors, a date that coups them in a stuffy hotel room probably won't put them in the most amorous of moods. The following section has his & her forget—me—not lists. Use the information to find out what your partner likes. There's nothing more romantic than finding out everything you can about one another and taking the time to make each other's needs and wants special.

It is not a matter of thinking a great deal but of loving a great deal, so do whatever arouses you most to love.

Saint Theresa of Avila

Forget me not my darling, for it is you
I adore.

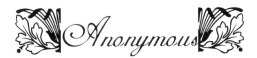
Anonymous

Forget Me Not List

Favorite type of gift(s) _____

Favorite flower(s) _____

Favorite song(s) _____

Favorite sport _____

Favorite type(s) of jewelry _____

Favorite color(s) _____

Favorite restaurant _____

Favorite drink/wine _____

Describe your

fantasy date _____

_____

_____

_____

Forget Me Not List

Favorite type of gift(s) _____

Favorite flower(s) _____

Favorite song(s)_____

Favorite sport _____

Favorite type(s) of jewelry_____

Favorite color(s)_____

Favorite restaurant _____

Favorite drink/wine _____

Describe your

fantasy date _____

_____

_____

_____

One of the oldest human needs is having someone to wonder where you are when you don't come home at night.

Margaret Mead

Love is the life of man.

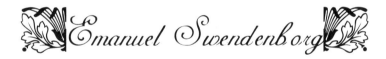

Emanuel Swendenborg

More Ways to Say
I Love You

One of the most romantic things we've ever seen on television happened on the Graham Kerr (formerly known as the Galloping Gourmet) show on the Discovery channel. He gave his wife, who had been his producer for many years a beautiful appreciation award. His words about her were very touching and he made a comment that we often give out awards in our business lives, but we forget to give awards to the people who mean the most to our lives. With that in mind, we've created a section of *Love Certificates & Love Coupons* for you to share with your mate.

Immediately following is the *Love Prescription* Section. This is a fun section that has some romantic prescriptions from the *Date Your Mate Paradise Clinic*. Copy these to share with each other & create some of your own.

Love Certificates

Love Certificate

This certifies that

_____

has been loving & caring throughout the year.

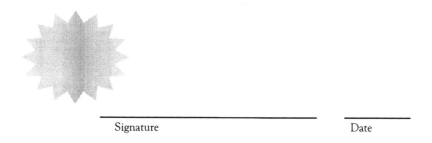

_____   _____
Signature   Date

Love Certificate

This certifies that

_____

is the world's greatest kisser.

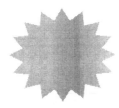

_____   _____
Signature   Date

Love Certificate

This certifies that

_____

is the most romantic person alive.

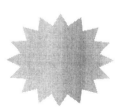

_____   _____

Signature   Date

Love Certificate

This certifies that

_____

has always loved me—even when I didn't love myself.

_____   _____

Signature   Date

Love Certificate

This certifies that

_____

is largely responsible for making my life complete.

_____   _____
Signature   Date

Love Certificate

This certifies that

_____

makes the world's best

_____

(fill in the blank)

_____   _____
Signature   Date

I like not only to be loved,

but to be told I am loved.

George Eliot

*L*ove that stammers,

that stutters, is apt to be the love that loves best.

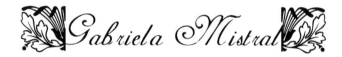
Gabriela Mistral

Love Coupons

~Love Coupon~

This coupon entitles bearer to a fantasy evening filled with fun, laughter & romance!

Compliments of:

_____

~Love Coupon~

Bearer of this coupon is entitled to one forgiveness
(1 promise)

Compliments of:

_____

~Love Coupon~

Bearer of this coupon is entitled to one $50.00 shopping spree at favorite lingerie store.

Compliments of:

_____

～Love Coupon～

Bearer of this coupon is entitled to one week off from doing household chores.

(This does include cooking *YES!*)

Compliments of:

_____

~Love Coupon~

Bearer of this coupon is entitled to one *entire weekend* of love & romance & me.

Compliments of:

_____

~Love Coupon~

This coupon entitles bearer to a candlelight dinner at a romantic restaurant.

Compliments of:

_____

~Love Coupon~

Bearer of this coupon is entitled to one **For Your Eyes Only** fashion show.

Compliments of:

_____

~Love Coupon~

One **Romantic Fantasy** fulfilled.

Compliments of:

_____

~Love Coupon~

This coupon is redeemable for 20 minutes of cuddling.

Compliments of:

_____

~Love Coupon~

Redeem this coupon at anytime for one breakfast in bed.

Compliments of:

_____

~Love Coupon~

Bearer of this coupon is entitled to one deeply personal & romantic love letter expressing exactly how your love makes me feel. (Please allow 2-3 days for redemption of this coupon)

Compliments of:

_____

~Love Coupon~

Redeemable for one fun evening of eating pizza and
watching your video of choice.

Compliments of:

_____

~Love Coupon~

Redeem this coupon to share a delectable hot fudge sundae (or dessert of choice) with me.

Compliments of:

_____

The cure for all the ills and wrongs, the cares, the sorrows, and the crimes of humanity, all lie in that one word "love." It is the divine vitality that everywhere produces and restores life. To each and every one of us, it gives the power of working miracles if we will.

Lydia Maria Child

Love is a little haven of rescue from the world.

Betrand A. Russell

Love Prescriptions

Date Your Mate Paradise Clinic

Address: Dr. S.O. GOOD
2-A Romantic Pl.   Dr. I..M. FUN
Love, ME 45683

FOR _____ DATE_____

R_x Apply 1 oz of lingerie & go straight to bed.

Label caution: May cause excitement & a rapid pulse.

☐ R_x can only be filled with your partner.

☐ May not substitute   Open: 24 hours a day 7 days a week

☐ Unlimited Refills _____ M.D.

Dispense as written

Date Your Mate Paradise Clinic

Address: Dr. S.O. RICHT
4 Sentiment Dr   Dr. I.N. LOVE
Cupids, Arrow 64523

FOR _____   DATE _____

R_x **Initial dose**: **Lingering hugs & kisses 1 x a day.**
Dosage may be increased based upon your response.

Label caution: May cause heightened pulse rate.

☐ **R**_x can only be filled with your partner.

☐ May not substitute   Open: 24 hours a day 7 days a week

☐ Unlimited Refills   _____ M.D.

Dispense as written

Date Your Mate Paradise Clinic

Address: Dr. PHOR EVER
24 Excitement.   Dr. DO. U. DATE
DATE, ME 47509

FOR ─────────────────────   DATE ─────────

R_x Perform moath to moath resuscitation on your partner.

Label caution: May cause a tingling sensation. Clinic is not responsible for

what may come next.

☐R_x can only be filled with your partner.

☐May not substitute   Open: 24 hours a day 7 days a week

☐Unlimited Refills   ──────────────────────── M.D.

Dispense as written

Date Your Mate Paradise Clinic

Address: Dr. D. D. DELIGHT
2-A Paradise Pl.   Dr. I. N. . CONTROL
I Love, YOU 45683

     FOR _____   DATE _____

R_x Put on sexy boxer shorts daily for one week followed by
a little exercise.

Label caution: May cause a heating sensation.

☐R_x can only be filled with your partner.

☐May not substitute   Open: 24 hours a day 7 days a week

☐Unlimited Refills _____ M.D.

Dispense as written

Date Your Mate Paradise Clinic

Address: Dr. D. O. RIGHT
2-4 A Date.   Dr. O. F. LOVE
Tonight's OK 45683

FOR _____   DATE _____

R_x Apply nothing on or in your mind. Lay back, relax and
enjoy a soothing massage.

Label caution: May increase heart rate & respiration's.

☐R_x can only be filled with your partner.

☐May not substitute   Open: 24 hours a day 7 days a week

☐Unlimited Refills

_____ M.D.

Dispense as written

Date Your Mate Paradise Clinic

Address: Dr. O. F. PASSION
2-4 A Date.   Dr. O.NE. LUV
Tonight's OK 45683

   FOR _____   DATE_____

R_x One weekend of loving, laughing & recharging our
        batteries at our favorite local hotel getaway.

Label caution: This prescription can be habit forming. Take as often as

needed.

☐R_x can only be filled with your partner.   Open: 24 hours a day 7 days a week

☐May not substitute   M.D.
                        _____
.☐Unlimited Refills

Dispense as written

Date Your Mate Paradise Clinic

Address: Dr. G. O. WILD
2-Lover's Lane   Dr. U. R. CUTE
Love, ME 45683

FOR _____ DATE _____

R_x Rab loving hands all over partner's back.

Label caution: May cause drowsiness. CAUTION! DO NOT OPERATE A

VEHICLE WHILE USING THIS PRESCRIPTION.

☐R_x can only be filled with your partner.

☐May not substitute   Open: 24 hours a day 7 days a week

☐Unlimited Refills   _____ M.D.

Dispense as written

∼ Order Form ∼

✂

❏ 101 Ways to Date Your Mate-
$7.95
❏ Sizzling Monogamy $12.95
❏ Romance Unlimited Catalog
(FREE)

☏ 505-899-3121
✉ **Mail Orders:**
W. H. Publishing—Dept2A.
4900 Mesa Bonita Ct. NW•
Albuquerque, NM 87120

Name: _____   Phone( ) _____

Address : _____

_____

Payment: ❏ Check ❏ Credit Card ❏ Money Order
(Make check/M.O. payable to: William Havens Publishing)
Credit Card Number: _____
Expiration Date: _____
Name on Card: _____

Shipping: $3.50 for 1st Book (add .50 for each additional)

Total $ Amount of items	Total Shipping Amount	**TOTAL**

We Want to Hear From YOU

Do you have a romantic story to tell? If you have a creative dating idea, please write to:

William Havens Publishing
4900 Mesa Bonita Ct. NW
Albuquerque, NM 87120

About the Authors

arl and Rose Smith, also know as *Mr. & Mrs. Romance*, have been happily married for eleven years and have been enjoying their marital affair for over eight years. Their affair started when Earl suggested they have a long distance love affair while he was serving his country overseas for a year. They live in Albuquerque, New Mexico with their two children.

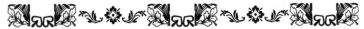